Time to try.....
the
BLOOD SUGAR
DIET

 CookNation

Time to try...the BLOOD SUGAR DIET

Quick & easy low carb, calorie counted recipes & quick start beginners guide

Disclaimer

CONTENTS

10 Great Soups 45

20 Delicious Dinners 57

5 Super Simple Desserts   79

10 Low Cal Smoothies   85

Other CookNation Titles   96

Time to try....
the
BLOOD SUGAR
DIET

INTRODUCTION

The Blood Sugar Diet is for anyone who has concerns about their blood sugar levels, wishes to lose weight in a healthy controlled manner and maintain a healthy diet for life.

It's time to try the Blood Sugar diet and enjoy the benefits of low carb, low sugar, low calorie recipes. Our delicious Time To Try calorie counted recipes will help bring your blood sugar back into the normal range; resulting in excess weight loss, lower levels of stress, increased energy and, if you already suffer from type 2 diabetes, you may also eventually become free of medication.

There are benefits to nearly everyone in following a low carb, low sugar diet however please consult with your doctor before embarking on a restricted calorie eating plan particularly if you have a pre-existing medical condition.

Raised Blood Sugar Levels

Abnormal levels of sugar in the blood can significantly increase the risks of a number of diseases and conditions including heart disease, type 2 diabetes, stroke, cancer & dementia.

Over a period of time a poor diet and not enough exercise can make your body less sensitive to insulin. Insulin is produced by the pancreas and one of it's main purposes is to bring high blood sugar levels down to the 'normal' range, diverting the energy from the glucose to the parts of the body that need it. If your body does become less sensitive to insulin and therefore blood sugar levels continue to rise, the pancreas continues producing insulin to counteract this BUT instead of being used up as energy it is stored as fat and so the cycle continues.

The Blood Sugar Diet

Time To Try The Blood Sugar Diet adheres to the basic diet principles of the Blood Sugar Diet by Michael Mosley. Michael Mosley's Blood Sugar Diet is a life changing approach to reducing blood sugar levels, reversing diabetes, losing weight and maintaining a healthy diet. We strongly recommend reading Dr. Mosley's book for an in-depth understanding of the problems of raised blood sugar levels. Our recipes have been written to complement this healthy approach to eating following a low carb, low calorie, Mediterranean style of cooking.

There are 3 ways to approach to the Blood Sugar Diet.

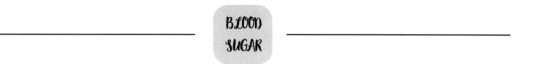

BLOOD
SUGAR

800 calorie 8 week fast:
This involves eating 800 calories every day of the week on a low carb Mediterranean 8 week fast.
This is the fastest way to lose weight and reduce blood sugar levels and should be maintained for up to 8 weeks.

A modified 5:2 Diet approach:
Follow a non calorie counted low carb Mediterranean diet for 5 days a week, and fast for 2 days a week with an 800 calorie fast for 2.

A non-calorie counted low carb, Mediterranean style diet:
This is a slower and lighter approach that is achieved by eating a non calorie counted low carb Mediterranean diet. Weight loss and blood sugar levels will take longer to fall but may be more suitable for those who do not wish to fast.

Please note; non-calorie counted doesn't mean you can eat as much as you like. It means you eat the 'normally' recommended calorie intake which is approx. 2500 calories per day for a man and 2000 for a woman.

The Principles Of The Mediterranean Style Blood Sugar Diet Plan

A Mediterranean diet is based on the healthy living habits of the populations of those countries bordering the Mediterranean Sea. It consists primarily of fresh vegetables, fruits, beans, whole grains, olive oil and fish. A Mediterranean Diet is a lifestyle choice rather than a strict list of what not to eat, it is a formula for daily healthy living.

Things to Avoid on The Blood Sugar Diet:

Avoid breakfast cereals
They are nearly all packed with sugar (even the 'healthy' ones).
Oats are a better alternative as they digest slowly keeping you feeling fuller for longer.

Avoid white carbs
They convert to sugar in your blood very quickly. White bread, potatoes, pasta and rice are all examples of white carbs. Brown or wholegrain alternatives, quinoa, bulgar wheat and buckwheat are better options.

Avoid sugar packed foods
No sugary drinks, sweets and desserts. Avoid too many tropical type fruits such as mango and pineapple which are high in natural sugar - even bananas!

Avoid Alcohol

It's packed with empty calories and won't help you lose weight. Although a glass of wine (preferably red) with a meal is acceptable.

Avoid snacking

Avoid snacks that are sweet and high in sugar. The sugar rush that follows quickly causes a sugar crash that makes us want to eat more. Healthier snack alternatives include nuts (not salted or coated in honey) or raw fresh veg like celery or carrot sticks. Dark chocolate (min 80% cocoa content) is also OK in small quantities.

Because the Blood Sugar Diet is low in carbs it allows us to eat a higher level of fat.

Healthy fats are good for us and give our bodies much needed energy. The advantage to using full fat dairy in your diet is that it keeps you feeling fuller for longer because they digest slowly and do not significantly increase blood sugar levels.

Dairy products however should be used in moderation due to their high level of calories. Trans-fats, which appear in processed foods, should be avoided at all costs. For cooking use olive, rapeseed or coconut oil.

About CookNation

CookNation is the leading publisher of innovative and practical recipe books for the modern, health conscious cook.

CookNation titles bring together delicious, easy and practical recipes with their unique approach - easy and delicious, no-nonsense recipes - making cooking for diets and healthy eating fast, simple and fun.

With a range of #1 best-selling titles - from the innovative 'Skinny' calorie-counted series, to the 5:2 Diet Recipes collection - CookNation recipe books prove that 'Diet' can still mean 'Delicious'!

Visit **www.bellmackenzie.com** to browse the full catalogue.

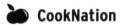 **CookNation**

10

Great Energy
BREAKFASTS

Portabella Avocado

366 calories per serving

Ingredients

- 2 tsp olive oil
- ½ garlic clove, crushed
- 1 large portabella mushroom
- 1 large beef tomato sliced

- 1 large free-range egg
- 1 avocado, stoned and sliced
- 1 baby gem lettuce shredded
- Salt & pepper to taste

Method

1 Preheat the oven grill.

2 Mix the oil and garlic together and brush over the underside of the mushroom.

3 Season well and place, underside up, under the grill for 5-7 minutes or until the mushroom is cooked through.

4 Meanwhile fill a pan with boiling water. Keep the boiling water gently simmering whilst you lower the egg into the pan to hard boil.

5 After 7 minutes peel the egg and cut in half.

6 Put the mushroom on the plate with the tomato slices. Arrange the lettuce over the top. Add the egg halves and pile over the avocado slices.

Chefs Note....
You could grill the tomato slices along with the mushroom if you wish.

Big Breakfast Frittata

375 calories per serving

Ingredients

- 1 tsp olive oil
- 3 shallots, chopped
- 5 sun dried tomatoes, chopped

- 50g/2oz feta cheese, crumbled
- 3 large free-range eggs
- 2 tbsp freshly chopped flat leaf parsley
- Salt & pepper to taste

Method

1 Heat the oil in a frying pan and gently sauté the shallots for a few minutes until softened.

2 Break the eggs into a bowl and combine with the feta cheese and sundried tomatoes. Tip the sautéed onions into the bowl along with the eggs.

3 Combine well and return the egg mixture to the pan, tilting to ensure the mixture covers the base evenly.

4 Cover the pan, reduce the heat and leave to cook for a few minutes. Flip the frittata over and cook the other side until the eggs set and the vegetables are tender.

5 Cut into wedges and serve with chopped parsley sprinkled over the top.

Chefs Note....
Add a little more feta cheese crumbled over the top to serve if you wish.

Quinoa & Messy Eggs

Ingredients

- 2 tsp olive oil
- ½ red onion, sliced
- 1 garlic clove, crushed
- 6 cherry tomatoes, halved
- 1 red pepper, deseeded & sliced
- 1 tsp paprika
- 50g/2oz cooked quinoa
- 2 large free-range eggs
- Salt & pepper to taste
- 1 tbsp chopped flat leaf parsley

Method

1 Gently heat the olive oil in a frying pan and sauté the onions, garlic, tomatoes and peppers for a few minutes until softened.

2 Add the paprika to the pan and stir. Cook for a minute or two longer before adding the eggs and quinoa to the pan.

3 Increase the heat, add seasoning and cook until the eggs are scrambled.

4 Check the seasoning & serve immediately. Garnish with chopped parsley.

Chefs Note....
Try adding some turmeric or garam masala for a spicy start to your day.

Avocado & Red Onion Salad

Ingredients

- ½ ripe avocado, peeled, stoned & cubed
- ½ red onion, sliced
- ½ tsp paprika
- 2 tsp lime juice
- 1 tsp extra virgin olive oil
- 1 tbsp freshly chopped coriander
- ½ cucumber
- 1 baby gem lettuce shredded
- Salt & pepper to taste

Method

1 Combine the cubed avocado, onion, paprika, lime, coriander, cucumber and lettuce together with the lime juice and olive oil.

2 Allow to sit for a few minutes to let the flavour infuse.

3 Season well and serve.

Chefs Note....

Stone the avocado by cutting in half (you'll need to work around the centre stone). When halved, dig the point of the knife into the stone to lever it out, then use a large spoon to scoop each half of the avocado out in one piece.

Blue Cheese Omelette

330 calories per serving

Ingredients

- 2 large free-range eggs
- 50g/5oz blue cheese, finely diced
- 1 tsp olive oil
- 1 tbsp freshly chopped chives
- 50g/2oz chopped spinach
- 75g/3oz cherry tomatoes, chopped
- Salt & pepper to taste

Method

1 Lightly beat the eggs with a fork. Season well and add the diced cheese, chives and spinach.

2 Gently heat the oil in a small frying pan and add the omelette mixture. Tilt the pan to ensure the mixture is evenly spread over the base.

3 Cook on a low to medium heat and, when the eggs are set underneath, fold the omelette in half and continue to cook for a further 2 minutes.

4 Serve with the chopped tomatoes sprinkled all over the top.

Chefs Note....
Check the eggs are set underneath by lifting with a fork before folding the omelette in half.

Blueberry Breakfast Smoothie

180 calories per serving

Ingredients

- 50g/2oz blueberries
- 50g/2oz spinach
- 250ml/1 cup soya milk

- 1 tsp flax seeds
- 1 tbsp vanilla Greek yogurt

Method

1 Rinse the blueberries and spinach and pat dry.

2 Remove any thick stalks from the spinach and give the flax seeds a bash with the rolling pin.

3 Blend all the ingredients together and serve immediately.

Chefs Note....
You could also add a handful of ice to this smoothie if you wish.

Paprika Eggs & Peppers

303 calories per serving

Ingredients

- 2 red peppers, deseeded & sliced
- 1 tsp paprika
- 2 large free-range eggs
- 2 tsp olive oil
- 50g/2oz watercress
- 1 tbsp freshly chopped coriander
- Salt & pepper to taste

Method

1 Break the eggs into a bowl. Add the paprika, lightly beat with a fork and season well.

2 Gently heat the oil in a frying pan and add the peppers. Sauté for a few minutes until they begin to soften.

3 Pour in the beaten eggs and move around the pan until the eggs begin to scramble. As soon as they start to set remove from the heat and serve with lots of black pepper, watercress and a sprinkle of fresh coriander.

Chefs Note....
Add a little chilli too if you want a kick to your morning.

Creamy Garlic Champignons

275 calories per serving

Ingredients

- 2 tsp olive oil
- 1 garlic clove, crushed
- ½ onion, sliced
- 150g/5oz mushrooms, sliced
- 2 tsp English mustard

- 2 tbsp crème fraiche
- 1 piece natural rye bread, lightly toasted
- 1 tbsp freshly chopped flat leaf parsley
- Pinch paprika
- Salt & pepper to taste

Method

1 Gently heat the oil in a pan and sauté the onions and garlic for a few minutes. Add the mushrooms and continue cooking for 8-10 minutes or until the mushrooms are soft and cooked through.

2 Stir through the mustard and crème fraiche, combine well and warm through.

3 Pile the creamy mushrooms and onions onto the rye toast.

4 Sprinkle with chopped parsley and paprika. Season and serve.

Chefs Note....
Mushrooms and garlic are a classic French combination great for breakfast.

Buckwheat & Matcha Pancakes

399 calories per serving

Ingredients

- 120ml/½ cup milk
- 1 medium free-range egg
- Pinch of salt
- 50g/2oz buckwheat flour
- 1 tsp matcha tea
- 50g/2oz strawberries
- 2 tsp butter
- 1 tbsp Greek yogurt

Method

1 Beat together the milk, egg and salt.

2 Place the buckwheat and matcha tea in another bowl.

3 Gradually add milk mixture to the flour and stir until you get a smooth batter.

4 Add the butter to a hot pan, pour in the mixture and cook for 1-2 minutes on each side, or until golden.

5 Remove from the pan and place to one side while you cook the others.

6 Serve with a dollop of yogurt and halved strawberries on top.

Chefs Note....
If you don't have matcha tea it's fine to omit this ingredient.

Walnut Yogurt

Ingredients

- 6 tbsp Greek Vanilla yogurt
- 1 tsp honey
- 10 walnut halves
- 125g/4oz blueberries

Method

1 Combine together the yogurt and honey.

2 Rinse the blueberries and finely chop the walnuts.

3 Sprinkle both onto the yogurt and serve.

Chefs Note....
According to new research walnuts can help at-risk adults reduce their chances of developing Type 2 diabetes.

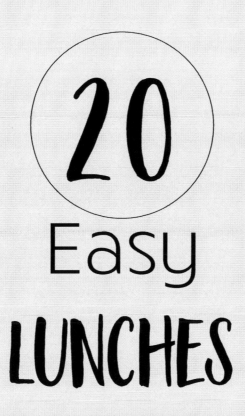

20 Easy

LUNCHES

Time to try....
the
BLOOD SUGER
DIET

Veg Italian Stew

Ingredients

- 2 tbsp olive oil
- 2 aubergines, cubed
- 1 red onion, chopped
- 2 celery stalk, chopped
- 1 garlic clove, crushed
- 2 tbsp balsamic vinegar

- 1 tsp capers, chopped
- 200g/3oz ripe tomatoes, roughly chopped
- 10 black pitted olives, sliced
- 2 tbsp freshly chopped parsley
- 50g/2oz Ricotta cheese
- Salt & pepper to taste

Method

1 Gently sauté the prepared aubergine, onions, celery and garlic in the olive oil for a few minutes until softened. Add the balsamic vinegar, capers, tomatoes & olives.

2 Stir, cover and continue to very gently cook for 20-25 minutes or until everything is cooked through and tender.

3 When the stew is ready stir through the ricotta, sprinkle with chopped parsley, season and serve.

Chefs Note....
You can also make this dish by slowly roasting in the oven with a splash of vegetable stock.

Roasted Ryvita Tomatoes

290 calories per serving

Ingredients

- 300g/10oz ripe plum tomatoes
- ½ tsp each dried thyme & oregano
- 1 tbsp olive oil
- 2 tbsp freshly chopped parsley
- 1 tbsp grated Parmesan
- 1 Ryvita
- Salt & pepper to taste

Method

1 Preheat the oven to 180C/350F/Gas4.

2 Halve the tomatoes and sprinkle with a little salt

3 Bash the Ryvita up to make breadcrumbs.

4 Place the tomatoes, dried herbs, olive oil, Parmesan and breadcrumbs in a bowl. Combine well and season.

5 Tip the tomatoes onto a grilling rack with a tray underneath to catch the juices. Place in the preheated oven and leave to cook for approx. 30-40 minutes.

6 Sprinkle with chopped parsley and serve.

Chefs Note....
This makes a great low carb lunch or a good side dish to a filling dinner.

Herb Couscous Salad

300 calories per serving

Ingredients

- 75g/5oz whole-wheat couscous
- 1 onion, chopped
- 2 garlic cloves, crushed
- 1 tbsp lime juice
- 1 tbsp olive oil
- 1 bunch spring onions, chopped

- Lime wedges to serve
- 2 tbsp freshly chopped mixed herbs
- 1 tbsp almonds, chopped
- 1 romaine lettuce, shredded
- Salt & pepper to taste

Method

1 Cook the couscous in salted boiling water for 6-8 minutes or until tender before draining.

2 Using a saucepan gently sauté the chopped onions & garlic for a few minutes.

3 Add the lime juice, fluff the couscous with a fork and pile into the onion pan.

4 Mix well, and serve over the shredded lettuce with fresh lime wedges on the side and the herbs & spring onions sprinkled over the top.

Chefs Note....
Also good as a dinner side dish with grilled chicken or tuna.

Borlotti & Prawn Salad Bowl

425 calories per serving

Ingredients

- 1 tbsp olive oil
- 3 shallots, sliced
- 1 garlic clove, crushed
- ½ red chilli, deseeded & finely chopped
- 8 cherry tomatoes, halved
- 200g/7oz tinned borlotti beans, drained
- 150g/5oz peeled raw king prawns
- 2 tsp lemon juice
- 1 tbsp freshly chopped basil
- 2 baby gem lettuce shredded
- Lemon wedges to serve
- Salt & pepper to taste

Method

1 Heat the olive in a pan and gently sauté the shallots, garlic & chilli for a few minutes until softened.

2 Add the tomatoes & beans and leave to gently simmer for 15 minutes stirring occasionally.

3 Add the prawns & lemon juice and combine well. Cover and simmer for a further 10 minutes or until the prawns are pink and cooked through.

4 Sprinkle with chopped basil and serve with lemon wedges and shredded lettuce.

Chefs Note....
Use whichever type of Italian bean you prefer for this recipe.

Triple Tomato Cod

390 calories per serving

Ingredients

- 1 tbsp olive oil
- 3 shallots, sliced
- 1 garlic clove, crushed
- 12 cherry tomatoes, chopped
- 120ml/½ cup tomato passata/sieved tomatoes
- 1 tbsp sundried tomato paste
- 10 pitted black olives, halved
- 1 tsp lemon juice
- 200g/7oz skinless, boneless cod fillets
- 1 tbsp freshly chopped basil
- Salt & pepper to taste

Method

1 Preheat the oven to 200C/400F/Gas Mark 6.

2 Gently sauté the shallots and garlic in the olive oil for a few minutes until softened. Add the chopped tomatoes, passata and sundried tomato paste and leave to gently simmer for 10 minutes stirring occasionally.

3 Add the olives & lemon juice and combine well to make a rich tomato sauce.

4 Place the fish fillets in an ovenproof dish and pour over the tomato sauce. Season well and place in the oven.

5 Cook for 20-30 minutes or until the fish is cooked through and piping hot. Sprinkle with chopped basil, season and serve.

Chefs Note....
As a serving idea pair with shredded steamed greens dressed in garlic and olive oil.

Broccoli & Bean Lunch Snack

265 calories per serving

Ingredients

- 2 tsp anchovy paste
- 200g/7oz tenderstem broccoli
- 150g/5oz soya beans
- 1 tbsp olive oil
- 2 garlic cloves, crushed
- 1 red onion, finely sliced
- 1 red chilli, deseeded & finely chopped
- Salt & pepper to taste

Method

1 Plunge the broccoli and soya beans into a pan of salted boiling water and cook for 2 minutes. Drain and put to one side.

2 Heat the olive oil in a frying pan and gently sauté the garlic, onion, chilli & anchovy paste and cook for a few minutes.

3 Add the broccoli and beans to the pan and increase the heat. Toss until well combined.

4 Check the seasoning and serve.

Chefs Note....
This recipe also works well with asparagus.

Pesto & Chicken Spirals

390 calories per serving

Ingredients

- 1 large courgette/zucchini
- 1 tsp extra virgin olive oil
- 150g/5oz chicken breast, sliced
- 1 tbsp pesto
- 2 shallots, sliced
- 2 tbsp freshly chopped flat leaf parsley
- 1 tbsp grated Parmesan cheese
- Salt & pepper to taste

Method

1 First spiralize the courgette into thick spirals.

2 Heat the olive oil in a high-sided frying pan and gently sauté the garlic and shallots for a few minutes.

3 Add the chicken and cook until piping hot and cooked through. Add the courgette spirals and increase the heat. Stir fry for 2-3 minutes and stir through the pesto.

4 Remove from the heat. Add the parsley and Parmesan.

5 Toss well, season & serve.

Chefs Note....
You will need a spiralizer for this dish if you don't have one pre-prepared shredded vegetables are now available in most supermarkets.

Truffle Oil 'Spaghetti'

290 calories per serving

Ingredients

- 1 large courgette/zucchini
- 125g/4oz mushrooms, sliced
- 1 tbsp truffle oil
- 1 garlic clove, crushed

- 1 onion, sliced
- 1 tbsp freshly chopped coriander
- 1 tbsp grated Parmesan cheese
- Salt & pepper to taste

Method

1 First spiralize the courgette into thin spaghetti noodles.

2 Heat the oil in a high-sided frying pan and gently sauté the mushrooms, garlic and onions for a few minutes until the mushrooms are cooked.

3 Add the courgette spaghetti and increase the heat.

4 Stir-fry for 2-3 minutes. Toss well, sprinkle with freshly chopped coriander and Parmesan. Season & serve.

Chefs Note....
You will need a spiralizer for this dish if you don't have one pre-prepared shredded vegetables are now available in most supermarkets.

Whole Meal Couscous Chicken

540 calories per serving

Ingredients

- 50g/2oz wholemeal couscous
- 500ml/2 cups vegetable stock
- 75g/3oz fresh peas
- 125g/4oz skinless chicken breast
- 3 shallots, chopped
- 1 tsp freshly grated ginger
- 1 garlic clove, crushed
- 1 tbsp olive oil
- Lemon wedges to serve
- 1 tbsp freshly chopped coriander
- Salt & pepper to taste

Method

1 Preheat the grill.

2 Cook the couscous in the boiling vegetable stock for 6-8 minutes or until tender. Drain and put to one side.

3 Meanwhile season the chicken breast. Grill for 15-20 mins or until cooked through and leave to cool before roughly chopping.

4 Gently sauté the chopped shallot, peas garlic & ginger in the olive oil for a few minutes and add the chicken.

5 Fluff the couscous with a fork and pile into the shallot pan. Mix well and serve with fresh lemon wedges on the side and chopped coriander sprinkled over the top.

Chefs Note....
Use frozen peas if you like but defrost before sautéing.

32

Mustard Salmon & Kale

380 calories per serving

Ingredients

- 150g/5oz skinless salmon fillet
- 75g/3oz kale, chopped
- 1 tbsp olive oil
- 1 garlic clove, crushed
- 1 tbsp freshly chopped chives

- 1 tbsp crème fraiche
- 2 tsp English mustard
- 2 tsp lemon juice
- Salt & pepper to taste

Method

1 Season the salmon fillet and place under a preheated grill for 10-12 minutes or until cooked through.

2 Meanwhile steam the kale for 8-10 minutes or until tender. Meanwhile heat the oil and garlic in a saucepan and gently sauté for a minute or two. Add the cooked kale, stir well and cook for a minute or two longer.

3 Gently combine together the chives, crème fraiche, mustard & lemon juice.

4 Arrange the salmon and sautéed kale on a plate. Pile the crème fraiche dressing on top. Season & serve.

Chefs Note....
A chicken fillet also works well for this simple lunchtime treat.

Tuna & Feta Salad

550 calories per serving

Ingredients

- 150g/5oz tinned tuna
- 10 cherry tomatoes
- 50g/2oz feta cheese
- 3 sundried tomatoes, finely chopped
- Handful pitted black olives
- ½ ripe avocado, peeled & stoned

- 2 tsp extra virgin olive oil
- 2 tsp cider vinegar
- 1 tbsp crème fraiche
- ½ tsp paprika
- 75g/3oz watercress
- Salt & pepper to taste

Method

1 Halve the cherry tomatoes and crumble the feta cheese.

2 Combine together the olive oil, vinegar, crème fraiche & paprika to make a dressing.

3 Toss the dressing, tomatoes, sundried tomatoes, cheese & avocado together in a large bowl and serve on a bed of watercress with the tuna and olives on top.

Chefs Note....
Dolcelatte cheese also works well in this recipe.

Asian Chicken Quinoa

580 calories per serving

Ingredients

- 150g/5oz skinless chicken breast, sliced
- 100g/3½oz soya beans
- 75g/3oz cooked quinoa
- 2 tsp olive oil
- 2 garlic cloves, crushed
- 1 onion, sliced

- 1 tsp grated fresh ginger
- 1 red chilli, de-seeded & finely chopped
- 200g/7oz spinach leaves, chopped
- 1 fresh lime wedge
- 1 tbsp cashew nuts, chopped
- Salt & pepper to taste

Method

1 Season the chicken.

2 Heat the olive oil in a frying pan and gently sauté the garlic, chilli, ginger and onions for a few minutes.

3 Add the chicken to the pan along with the soya beans. Stir-fry for 8-10 minutes until the chicken is cooked through then add the quinoa along with the spinach.

4 Combine for a minute or two, pile into a bowl with the nuts sprinkled over the top and the lime wedge on the side. Check the seasoning and serve.

Chefs Note....
Quinoa is an excellent option for the blood sugar diet with its whole-grain and low glycemic index properties.

Blue Cheese Steak

540 calories per serving

Ingredients

- 150g/5oz beef steak
- 1 tbsp olive oil
- ½ red onion, sliced
- ½ garlic clove, crushed
- 2 red peppers, deseeded & sliced
- 10 cherry tomatoes, halved
- Handful of baby spinach
- 50g/2oz blue cheese, cubed
- Salt & pepper to taste

Method

1 Lightly brush the steak with a little of the olive oil. Season and put a frying pan on a high heat.

2 In another pan gently sauté the peppers, onions & garlic in the rest of the olive oil for 5-7 minutes or until tender.

3 Place the steak in the smoking hot dry pan and cook for 2 minutes each side, or to your liking.

4 Whilst the steak is cooking add the spinach and blue cheese to the pan of vegetables. Stir through until the spinach wilts and the cheese melts.

5 Place the steak on a plate and pile everything else on top. Season and serve.

Chefs Note....
As an alternative you could use pork tenderloin for this recipe. Make sure the pork is cooked though before serving.

Tuna & Balsamic Tomatoes

350 calories per serving

Ingredients

- 6 vine ripened tomatoes, chopped
- ½ red onion, finely chopped
- 1 tbsp chopped basil
- 1 tbsp balsamic vinegar
- 2 tsp olive oil
- 1 fresh tuna steak, weighing 150g/5oz
- 75g/3oz mixed salad
- Salt & pepper to taste

Method

1 Gently combine the tomatoes and red onion in 1 teaspoon of the olive oil and the balsamic vinegar along with the chopped basil.

2 Season the tuna. Put a frying pan on a high heat with the rest of the olive oil.

3 Place the tuna in the pan and cook for 2 minutes each side. Remove the tuna from the pan and serve with the salad on the side and the dressed tomatoes piled on top.

Chefs Note....
Two minutes of cooking each side should leave the tuna rare in the centre. Reduce or increase cooking time depending on your preference.

Chilli & Lime Cobbler

420 calories per serving

Ingredients

- 1 tsp lime juice
- 1 tsp grate fresh ginger
- ½ red chilli, de-seeded & finely chopped
- 6 cherry tomatoes, diced
- 1 spring onions, finely chopped
- ½ avocado, peeled & stoned

- 1 garlic clove, crushed
- 2 tsp olive oil
- 1 boneless, skinless cobbler fillet weighing 150g/5oz
- 50g/2oz watercress
- Salt & pepper to taste

Method

1 Preheat the grill.

2 Combine together the lime juice, ginger, chilli, cherry tomatoes, spring onions and avocado to create a chunky salad.

3 Mix together the garlic & olive oil and brush onto the cobbler fillet.

4 Place the fish under the preheated grill and cook for 6-9 minutes or until the fillet is cooked through.

5 Season and serve the fish with the salad over the top and the watercress on the side of the plate.

Chefs Note....
Use cobbler fillets or any other firm white fish.

Sardine Spinach Salad

395 calories per serving

Ingredients

- 2 x 100g (3 1/2oz) sardines,
- 2 tsp curry powder
- 1 tsp olive oil
- 1 tbsp mayonnaise
- 1 tsp lemon juice
- 1 tsp Tabasco sauce
- 100g/3½oz spinach
- Salt & pepper to taste

Method

1 Season the sardines and rub with the curry powder.

2 Heat the olive oil in a pan and fry the fillets for 3 minutes each side.

3 Meanwhile combine together the mayonnaise, lemon juice & Tabasco to make a dressing.

4 When the fish is cooked, wrap in foil and put to one side to keep warm. Add the spinach to the empty pan and cook for a few minutes.

5 Remove from the heat, stir the dressing through the wilted spinach and serve with the cooked sardine fillets.

Chefs Note....
Spinach and sardines make an unbeatable superfood combination.

Pesto Salmon & Lentils

420 calories per serving

Ingredients

- 200g/7oz tinned lentils
- 1 boneless, skinless salmon fillet weighing 150g/5oz
- 2 tsp grated Parmesan cheese
- 1 tsp pesto
- Lemon wedges to serve
- Salt & pepper to taste

Method

1 Season the salmon fillet. Mix the Parmesan cheese and pesto together and coat the top of the salmon fillet with the pesto mixture.

2 Place the salmon under a preheated grill and cook for 10-13 minutes or until the salmon fillet is cooked through.

3 Whilst the salmon is cooking warm the lentils.

4 When the salmon is ready lay the cooked fillet on top of the cooked noodles and squeeze lemon juice over the top.

Chefs Note....
Tinned lentils are a great store cupboard ingredient. They are a low GI food and are packed with protein.

Walnut & Kale Snack Lunch

285 calories per serving

Ingredients

- 150g/5oz Kale
- 2 tsp butter
- 1 onion, chopped
- 6 walnuts finely chopped

- ½ tsp turmeric
- A drizzle of extra virgin olive oil
- Salt & pepper to taste

Method

1 Shred the kale, removing any thick stalks.

2 Heat the butter in a frying pan and gently sauté the onion and walnuts with the turmeric for a few minutes until the onions are soft and golden.

3 Add the kale and continue to sauté until the kale is tender.

4 Season with plenty of salt & freshly ground pepper and a drizzle of olive oil.

Chefs Note....
Pine nuts also work well in this simple lunchtime snack.

Crab Chickpea Salad

520 calories per serving

Ingredients

- ½ cucumber, finely diced
- ½ tsp honey
- 2 tsp rice wine vinegar
- Pinch dried chilli flakes
- ½ red onion, finely chopped
- 200g/7oz tinned chickpeas, drained & rinsed
- 3 vine ripened tomatoes, chopped
- 150g/5oz tinned crabmeat, drained
- ½ avocado, cubed
- 1 baby gem lettuce, shredded
- Salt & pepper to taste

Method

1 Combine together the cucumber, rice wine vinegar, honey & chilli flakes.

2 Add the red onion, chickpeas, tomatoes, crabmeat, avocado and lettuce to make a tasty salad.

3 Season and serve.

Chefs Note....
steamed green beans also make a good addition to this simple salad.

Tabasco Shrimp Cocktail

395 calories per serving

Ingredients

- 1 tbsp mayonnaise
- 1 tsp Tabasco sauce
- ½ tsp lemon juice
- 1 tsp freshly chopped chives
- 200g/7oz cooked & peeled prawns

- 6 vine ripened tomatoes, diced
- ½ cucumber, diced
- Handful of watercress
- ½ ripe avocado, peeled, stoned & diced
- Salt & pepper to taste

Method

1 Mix together the mayonnaise, Tabasco sauce, lemon juice, chives, prawns, cucumber, avocado and tomatoes until everything is combined.

2 Place the watercress in and shallow bowl. Pile the dressed prawns on top and serve.

Chefs Note....
Sprinkle with a little paprika and serve with lemon wedges.

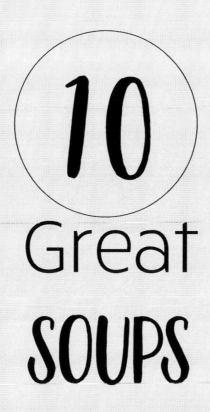

10
Great
SOUPS

Time to try....
the
BLOOD SUGER
DIET

Creamy Broccoli & Stilton Soup

290 calories per serving

Ingredients

- 1 tbsp olive oil
- 4 shallots, chopped
- 1 garlic clove, crushed
- 50g/2oz wild rice
- 500g/1lb 2oz broccoli florets

- 1lt/4 cups vegetable or chicken stock
- 2 tbsp crème fraiche
- 125g/4oz Stilton cheese, finely chopped
- Salt & pepper to taste

Method

1 Gently heat the olive oil in a large non-stick saucepan and add the shallots & garlic.

2 Sauté for a few minutes until the shallots soften.

3 Add the wild rice, broccoli florets & stock and simmer for 12-16 minutes or until the rice is tender.

4 Tip the soup into a blender or food processor, along with the crème fraiche, and whizz until you have a completely smooth texture.

5 Stir through the Stilton cheese. Check the seasoning and serve.

Chefs Note....
Use mild onions if you don't have shallots to hand.

Carrot & Double Coriander Soup

165 calories per serving

Ingredients

- 1 tbsp olive oil
- 1 onion, sliced
- 2 garlic cloves, crushed
- 600g/1lb 5oz carrots, peeled & chopped
- 1 tsp ground coriander/cilantro
- 1lt/4 cups vegetable or chicken stock
- 4 tbsp single cream
- 4 tbsp freshly chopped coriander/cilantro
- Salt & pepper to taste

Method

1 Gently sauté the onions & garlic with the olive oil in a large non-stick saucepan for a few minutes until softened.

2 Add the carrots, ground coriander & stock and simmer for 8-12 minutes or until the carrots are tender.

3 Tip the soup into a blender or food processor and whizz until you have a completely smooth texture.

4 Check the seasoning, swirl a tablespoon of cream through each bowl of soup and sprinkle with freshly chopped coriander.

Chefs Note....
Add a little more stock to alter the consistency of the soup if you wish.

Chicken Broth

170 calories per serving

Ingredients

- 2 onions, sliced
- 3 celery stalks, chopped
- 200g/7oz carrots, peeled & chopped
- 3 garlic cloves, crushed
- 2 bay leaves
- 1 tbsp white peppercorns

- 2 tbsp freshly chopped flat leaf parsley
- 300g/11oz chicken breast (leave the breast whole)
- 1.25lt/5 cups vegetable or chicken stock
- Salt & pepper to taste

Method

1 Add all the ingredients to a large non-stick saucepan, bring to the boil and simmer for 15-20 minutes or until the chicken is cooked through.

2 Remove the chicken breast and put to one side.

3 Meanwhile pass the soup through a sieve to create a clear broth. Return the soup to the pan and place on a gentle heat.

4 Use two forks to shred the chicken breast. Add the shredded chicken back to the pan and warm through for a few minutes.

5 Check the seasoning and serve.

Chefs Note....
This is a simple clear broth. Perfect for a light lunch on wintry days.

Pea & Yogurt Soup

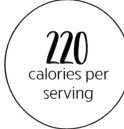

220 calories per serving

Ingredients

- 1 tbsp olive oil
- 1 onion, sliced
- 2 sticks of celery
- 2 garlic cloves, crushed
- ½ tsp dried thyme
- 1lt/4 cups vegetable or chicken stock
- 50g/2oz wild rice
- 500g/1lb 2oz peas
- 4 tbsp Greek yogurt
- ½ tsp paprika
- Salt & pepper to taste

Method

1 Gently sauté the olive oil, onions, celery, garlic & thyme in a large non-stick saucepan for a few minutes until softened.

2 Add the stock & wild rice and simmer for 10 minutes. Add the peas and continue to cook until the rice is tender.

3 Tip the soup into a blender or food processor and whizz until you have a completely smooth texture.

4 Check the seasoning and serve with a tablespoon of Greek yogurt swirled though the soup, sprinkle with paprika and serve.

Chefs Note....
Also good with broad beans or soya beans in the place of peas.

Beetroot & Horseradish Soup

165 calories per serving

Ingredients

- 1 tbsp olive oil
- 1 onion, sliced
- 600g/1lb 5oz cooked beetroot, chopped
- 1lt/4 cups vegetable or chicken stock
- 4 tbsp Greek yogurt
- 1 tbsp horseradish sauce
- Salt & pepper to taste

Method

1 Gently heat the olive oil in a large non-stick saucepan and sauté the onions for a few minutes until softened.

2 Add the beetroot & stock and simmer for 5-6 minutes or until everything is cooked through and piping hot.

3 Tip the soup into a blender or food processor along with the yogurt & horseradish sauce and whizz until you have a completely smooth texture.

4 Check the seasoning and serve.

Chefs Note....
Adjust the quantity of horseradish to suit your own taste.

Super Spinach Soup

289 calories per serving

Ingredients

- 1 tbsp olive oil
- 5 shallots, sliced
- 2 celery stalks, chopped
- 125g/4oz peas
- 150g/5oz spinach
- 1lt/4 cups vegetable stock
- 120ml/½ cup single cream
- Salt & pepper to taste

Method

1 Heat a pan and gently sauté the shallots and celery in the olive oil for a few minutes.

2 Add all the other ingredients, except the cream, to the pan.

3 Bring to the boil, cover and leave to gently simmer for 8-10 minutes or until everything is tender. Blend to your preferred consistency stir through the cream, season and serve immediately.

Chefs Note....
Try serving with some finely chopped walnuts sprinkled over the top.

Cannellini Soup

Ingredients

- 1 tbsp olive oil
- 2 garlic cloves, crushed
- 2 shallots, chopped
- 1lt/4cups vegetable stock

- Large bunch basil, chopped
- 400g/14oz tinned cannellini
- 125ml/½ cup single cream
- Salt & pepper to taste

Method

1 Gently sauté the shallots and garlic in the olive oil for a few minutes.

2 Add all the ingredients, except the cream, to the pan.

3 Bring to the boil, cover and leave to simmer for 10-15 minutes or until everything is tender.

4 Blend to your preferred consistency, season and serve with the cream stirred through.

Chefs Note....
Use whichever white Italian bean you prefer for this filling soup, store extra portions in the fridge or freezer.

Lentil & Pumpkin Seed Soup

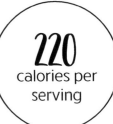

220 calories per serving

Ingredients

- 400g/14oz tinned green lentils
- 4 shallots, chopped
- 2 garlic cloves, crushed
- 4 tbsp chopped flat leaf parsley
- 1lt/4 cups vegetable stock/broth
- 120ml/½ cup milk
- 2 tbsp pumpkin seeds, chopped
- Salt & pepper to taste

Method

1 Add all the ingredients, except the milk, pumpkin seeds, to the saucepan.

2 Bring to the boil and leave to gently simmer for 8-10 minutes.

3 Blend to a smooth consistency, add the milk, and heat through for a minute or two.

4 Check the seasoning and serve with freshly chopped parsley and pumpkin seeds sprinkled over the top.

Chefs Note....
Cooked lentils are widely available and are a great time saver.

Creamy Asparagus & Hazelnut Soup

180 calories per serving

Ingredients

- 2 tsp butter
- 2 garlic cloves, crushed
- 4 shallots, sliced
- 300g/10oz asparagus, chopped

- 1lt/4 cups vegetable stock/broth
- 120ml/½ cup single cream
- 1 tbsp roasted hazelnuts, chopped
- Salt & pepper to taste

Method

1 Heat the butter and gently sauté the garlic, shallots and asparagus for a few minutes until softened.

2 Add all the ingredients, except the cream and hazelnuts, to a saucepan. Bring to the boil and simmer for 5 minutes or until tender.

3 Blend the soup well in the food processor.

4 Check the seasoning, stir through the cream, sprinkle over the hazelnuts and serve immediately.

Chefs Note....
Creamy and nutritious, this soup is a great lunchtime option.

Chilled Summer Soup

175 calories per serving

Ingredients

- 1 tbsp olive oil
- 4 shallots, sliced
- 2 garlic cloves, crushed
- 800g/1¾lb peas

- 1 iceberg lettuce, roughly chopped
- 1.25lt/5 cups vegetable or chicken stock
- 2 tbsp freshly chopped mint
- Salt & pepper to taste

Method

1 Gently heat the olive oil in a large non-stick saucepan, add the shallots & garlic and sauté for a few minutes until softened.

2 Add the peas, lettuce, stock & mint and simmer for 3-5 minutes or until the peas are cooked through and everything is piping hot.

3 Tip the soup into a blender or food processor and whizz until you have a completely smooth texture.

4 Place in a large bowl, cover and leave to cool. When it's cool place in the refrigerator to chill.

5 Serve in shallow bowls with plenty of black pepper.

Chefs Note....
A swirl of cream makes a good addition to this unusual and refreshing chilled soup.

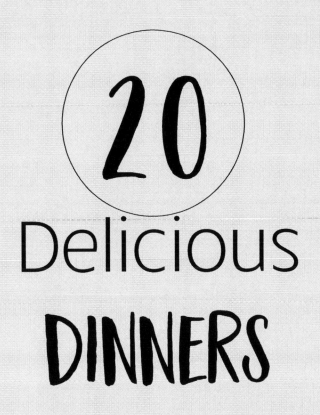

20 Delicious DINNERS

Italian Chicken

540 calories per serving

Ingredients

- 150g/5oz chicken breast
- ½ red onion, thickly sliced
- 2 tsp green pesto
- 50g/5oz chopped spinach

- 75g/3oz wild rice
- 500ml/2 cups vegetable stock
- 1 tsp olive oil
- Salt & pepper to taste

Method

1 Preheat the oven to 200C/400F/gas Mark 6

2 Hold the chicken breast as if you were slicing through the centre of it. Stop slicing before you cut it in half completely (this will butterfly the breast). Open the chicken breast to expose the two inside parts. Spread the inside of each breast with the pesto and close the 'sandwich' back up so you are left with pesto through the centre of the chicken breast. Place the chicken, on a baking tray, season well, brush with olive oil and cover with foil.

3 Place in the oven and leave to cook for 25-30 minutes or until the chicken is cooked through.

4 Meanwhile cook the wild rice in boiling vegetable stock (add a little more if needed). When it is ready drain and stir the chopped spinach through.

5 Season and serve the spinach wild rice and chicken together.

Chefs Note....
Also good with a crisp green salad.

Greek Pork Kebabs

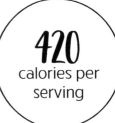

420 calories per serving

Ingredients

- ½ garlic clove, crushed
- 1 tbsp olive oil
- 150g/5oz pork tenderloin, cubed
- 1 tbsp Greek yoghurt
- 2 tsp paprika
- 1 red pepper, deseeded & cut onto chunks
- 1 red onion, peeled and cut into chunks
- 8 button mushrooms
- 2 tbsp freshly chopped coriander
- Salt & pepper to taste
- Metal skewers

Method

1 Preheat the grill to a medium/high heat.

2 Mix together the garlic, olive oil, yoghurt and paprika in a bowl.

3 Season the pork and add to the oil. Combine well and skewer each piece of pork and vegetable in turn to make two pork and vegetable kebabs.

4 Place under the grill and cook for 6-8 minutes each side or until the pork is cooked through and piping hot.

5 Remove from the grill, season and serve with chopped coriander sprinkled over the top.

Chefs Note....
Substitute the coriander with basil if preferred.

Minted Halloumi

460 calories per serving

Ingredients

- 75g/3oz sliced halloumi
- 2 shallots onion, chopped
- 75g/3oz fresh peas
- ½ garlic clove, crushed
- 1 red pepper, deseeded & finely chopped
- 2 tsp olive oil
- 75g/3oz whole wheat giant couscous
- 2 tbsp freshly chopped mint
- Salt & pepper to taste

Method

1 Cook the couscous in salted boiling water for 6-8 minutes or until tender.

2 Meanwhile gently sauté the chopped shallots, peas, garlic & peppers in the olive oil until softened.

3 In a separate pan add the halloumi. You don't need to use any oil. Cook the first side of the halloumi for a minute or two. Flip and cook for a further minutes.

4 Drain the couscous and fluff with a fork. Combine in the pan with the peppers and onions.

5 Pile into a shallow bowl. Sit the halloumi on top, sprinkle with parsley and serve.

Chefs Note....
Feel free to use frozen peas but defrost them first.

Feta Asparagus

390 calories per serving

Ingredients

- 250g/9oz asparagus spears
- 1 tbsp olive oil
- 1 tsp balsamic vinegar

- 2 slices Parma ham
- 75g/3oz feta cheese, crumbled
- Salt & pepper to taste

Method

1 Preheat the grill to a medium/high heat.

2 In a bowl mix together the asparagus, oil and vinegar ensuring each asparagus spear is coated with oil.

3 Place under the grill and cook for 4-6 minutes each side or until cooked through.

4 Remove from the grill, season and serve immediately with the Parma ham laid over the asparagus and the feta crumbled on top.

Chefs Note....
Feel free to replace Parma ham with some finely chopped sundried tomatoes.

Garlic Mussels

410
calories per
serving

Ingredients

- 500g/1lb 2oz mussels
- 2 tbsp olive oil
- 3 garlic cloves, crushed
- 3 shallots, sliced
- 200g/7oz tinned chopped tomatoes
- 60ml/¼ cup vegetable stock
- 2 tbsp freshly chopped basil
- Salt & pepper to taste

Method

1 Make sure the mussels are cleaned to rid them of any debris or seaweed.

2 Place in a colander and rinse thoroughly under running water.

3 Heat the oil in a large lidded pan and gently sauté the garlic and shallots.

4 After a few minutes increase the heat and add the chopped tomatoes and vegetable stock.

5 Place the mussels in the pan, cover with the lid and steam, for approximately 4-5 minutes, shaking the pan occasionally.

6 Tip the mussels and sauce into a shallow bowl. Sprinkle with basil and serve.

Chefs Note....
Discard any mussels that remain shut after cooking. These should not be eaten.

Simply Grilled Tuna

430 calories per serving

Ingredients

- 1 fresh tuna steak weighing 175g/6oz
- 1 tbsp extra virgin olive oil
- 2 tsp lemon juice
- 1 tbsp freshly chopped basil
- 75g/3oz watercress
- 125g/3oz vine ripened tomatoes, sliced
- 1 tbsp Parmesan shavings
- Lemon wedges to serve
- Salt & pepper to taste

Method

1 Preheat the grill to a medium/high heat.

2 Mix together the olive oil and lemon juice and lightly brush on either side of the steak (reserving any remaining juice).

3 Place the tuna steak under the grill and cook for 2-3 minutes each side or until the tuna is cooked to your liking.

4 Remove from the grill, season and place on a plate with the watercress and tomatoes. Drizzle any remaining juice over the top along with the Parmesan shavings and fresh basil. Serve with the lemon wedges.

Chefs Note....
Fresh tuna is best served rare in the centre, but feel free to adjust to your own taste.

Tasty Herbed Lentils

410 calories per serving

Ingredients

- 200g/7oz cooked tinned lentils
- 200g/7oz peas
- 2 tsp olive oil
- 3 anchovy fillets, drained
- ½ garlic clove, crushed
- 2 shallots, sliced
- 100g/3½oz ripe plum tomatoes, roughly chopped
- 2 tbsp freshly chopped mint & basil
- 50g/2oz rocket
- Salt & pepper to taste

Method

1 Place the peas in a pan of boiling water, cook for 2 minutes and drain.

2 Meanwhile heat the olive oil in a high-sided frying pan and gently sauté the anchovy fillets, garlic, onions and chopped tomatoes. Once cooked, leave to cool.

3 Drain the lentils and toss well with the cooled tomato mix.

4 Pile onto top of a bed or rocket and serve with the chopped fresh herbs over the top.

Chefs Note....
Try garnishing this with some extra fresh tomatoes, raw red onions and cubed avocado.

Veg Quinoa Salad

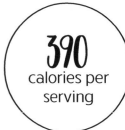

390
calories per
serving

Ingredients

- 75g/3oz quinoa
- 500ml/2 cups vegetable stock
- 2 tsp olive oil
- ½ garlic clove, crushed
- 1 red pepper, sliced
- ½ aubergine, cubed

- ½ red onion, chopped
- 75g/3oz cherry tomatoes, halved
- 50g/2oz spinach leaves
- 50g/2oz feta cheese
- 3 sundried tomatoes, chopped
- Salt & pepper to taste

Method

1 Cook the quinoa in vegetable stock (adding more if needed). When it's tender drain and put to one side.

2 Mix the olive oil, garlic, peppers, aubergine, onions and tomatoes in a bowl. Add to a frying pan and gently sauté for 10 minutes or until all the vegetables are tender and cooked through.

3 Add the cooked quinoa to the pan and combine well. Pile everything on a plate on top of the spinach, crumble over the feta cheese. Season and serve.

Chefs Note....
Use sundried tomatoes from a jar as they are nice and soft and perfect for salads.

Tropical Chicken Skewers

360 calories per serving

Ingredients

- 1 garlic clove, crushed
- 1 tbsp extra virgin olive oil
- 2 tsp lemon juice
- 150g/5oz chicken breast, cubed
- 75g/3oz pineapple chunks
- 1 red pepper, cut into chunks
- Handful of cherry tomatoes
- Salt & pepper to taste
- Metal skewers

Method

1 Preheat the grill to a medium/high heat.

2 Mix together the garlic, olive oil & lemon juice in a bowl.

3 Add the chicken, peppers, cherry tomatoes & pineapple pieces and season.

4 Combine well and skewer each piece in turn to make two large kebabs.

5 Place under the grill and cook for 6-8 minutes each side or until the chicken is cooked through.

6 Remove from the grill, season and serve.

Chefs Note....
These skewers are great served with mixed salad and a dollop of Greek yoghurt.

Grilled Cod & Mozzarella

SERVES 1

380 calories per serving

Ingredients

- 150g/5oz skinless, boneless cod fillet
- 1 garlic clove, crushed
- 1 tbsp extra virgin olive oil
- 2 tsp lemon juice
- 1 tbsp freshly chopped mint

- 2 large ripe beef tomatoes, thickly sliced
- 50g/2oz mozzarella cheese, sliced
- 75g/2oz mixed salad leaves
- Salt & pepper to taste

Method

1 Preheat the grill to a medium/high heat.

2 Mix together the garlic, olive oil & lemon juice and brush on either side of the fish fillet and tomatoes. Place the fish and tomatoes under the grill and cook for 2-3 minutes each side or until the cod is cooked through.

3 Lay the tomatoes on top of the fish and sit the mozzarella slices on top. Place back under the grill until the mozzarella is melted and bubbles.

4 Sit the cooked fish on the plate to the side of the salad leaves and sprinkle the mint all over.

Chefs Note....
Use whichever fish you prefer.
Firm white fish is best.

Olive & Asparagus Quinoa

345 calories per serving

Ingredients

- 75g/3oz quinoa
- 500ml/2 cups vegetable stock
- 125g/4oz asparagus tips
- 8 pitted black olives, sliced
- ½ onion, chopped
- 1 garlic clove, crushed

- 1 tbsp lemon juice
- 2 tsp olive oil
- Lemon wedges to serve
- 1 tbsp freshly chopped mint
- Salt & pepper to taste

Method

1 Cook the quinoa in boiling stock for 15 minutes or until tender. (Add a little more stock if needed.)

2 Gently sauté the sliced olives, chopped onions, garlic, lemon juice and asparagus in the olive oil for a few minutes.

3 When the quinoa is ready drain off any excess liquid. Fluff with a fork and pile into the onion and asparagus pan.

4 Mix well and serve with fresh lemon wedges on the side and chopped mint sprinkled over the top.

Chefs Note....
You could use chopped basil or coriander in place of mint if you like.

Brown Rice & Caper Stir Fry

380 calories per serving

Ingredients

- 75g/3oz brown rice
- 750ml/3 cups vegetable stock
- 200g/7oz ripe cherry tomatoes
- 1 tbsp capers
- 1 tbsp sultanas

- 2 tsp olive oil
- ½ garlic clove, crushed
- 3 sundried tomatoes (from a jar)
- 1 tbsp freshly chopped basil
- Salt & pepper to taste

Method

1 Cook the brown rice in boiling stock for about 15 minutes or until it's tender. (Add a little more stock if needed).

2 Meanwhile half the cherry tomatoes and roughly chop the capers, sultanas and sundried tomatoes.

3 Heat the olive oil and gently sauté the garlic, cherry tomatoes, capers, sultanas and sundried tomatoes whilst the rice cooks.

4 When the rice is ready drain any excess water and add to the frying pan.

5 Toss well and serve with chopped basil on top.

Chefs Note....
This is also good served with cauliflower rice in place of brown rice.

Garlic Prawns

315 calories per serving

Ingredients

- 1 tbsp butter
- 3 garlic cloves, crushed
- 4 shallots, sliced
- 250g/9oz raw, shelled king prawns

- 2 tbsp freshly chopped flat leaf parsley
- 1 lemon wedge
- 2 romaine lettuces shredded
- Salt & pepper to taste

Method

1 Heat the butter in a saucepan and gently sauté the garlic, shallots & prawns.

2 Toss well. Arrange the shredded lettuce in a shallow bowl and pile the prawns and shallots on top.

3 Sprinkle with chopped parsley, a squeeze of lemon and serve.

Chefs Note....
Prawns, lemon and garlic are a match made in heaven. Add more garlic if you prefer a stronger taste.

Salmon & Fennel

440 calories per serving

Ingredients

- 50g/2oz brown rice
- 2 tsp olive oil
- ½ onion, sliced
- ½ fennel bulb, finely sliced
- 1 garlic clove, crushed
- 200g/7oz ripe plum tomatoes, roughly chopped
- 60ml/¼ cup vegetable or chicken stock/broth
- 150g/5oz skinless, boneless salmon fillet
- Lemon wedges to serve
- 1 tbsp freshly chopped flat leaf parsley
- Salt & pepper to taste

Method

1 Cook the rice in salted boiling water until tender then drain.

2 In a shallow saucepan gently sauté the onion, fennel & garlic in the olive oil for a few minutes until softened.

3 Add the roughly chopped tomatoes & stock and leave to gently simmer for 10 minutes stirring occasionally.

4 Add the fish fillet and gently combine well. Cover and simmer for a further 8-10 minutes or until the fish is cooked through and the sauce has reduced.

5 Add the drained rice and combine well.

6 Season well and serve with lemon wedges and parsley sprinkled over the top.

Chefs Note....
To keep the salmon fillet whole you could grill it separately and serve over the tomato, rice and fennel sauce when it's ready.

Basil Chicken

496 calories per serving

Ingredients

- 2 tsp olive oil
- 3 shallots, sliced
- ½ fennel bulb, finely sliced
- 1 garlic cloves, crushed
- 200g/7oz tinned flageolet beans, drained
- 150g/5oz skinless chicken breasts, thickly sliced
- 60ml/¼ cup chicken stock/broth
- 125g/4oz spinach
- 2 tbsp freshly chopped basil
- 2 tsp Parmesan shavings
- Salt & pepper to taste

Method

1 Gently sauté the shallots, fennel and garlic in the olive oil for a few minutes until softened.

2 Add the beans, chicken & stock and leave to gently simmer for 10-15 minutes or until the chicken is cooked through and the stock has reduced.

3 Stir through the spinach until wilted.

4 Sprinkle with chopped basil and Parmesan shaving. Season and serve.

Chefs Note....
Parmesan and fennel are a classic Italian combination.

Pork & Beans

410 calories per serving

Ingredients

- 2 tsp olive oil
- ½ red onion, sliced
- 1 tsp freshly grated ginger
- ½ garlic clove, crushed
- 1 celery stalk, chopped
- 150g/5oz pork tenderloin, cubed
- 1 tbsp fresh chopped marjoram
- 60ml/¼ cup chicken stock/broth
- 75g/3oz fresh edamame beans
- 125g/4oz spinach leaves
- Salt & pepper to taste

Method

1 In a saucepan gently sauté the onion, celery, ginger and garlic in the olive oil for a few minutes until softened.

2 Add the pork, marjoram & stock and leave to gently simmer for 8-10 minutes or until the pork is cooked through and the stock has reduced.

3 Add the edamame beans and cook for a minute or two. Add the spinach and stir for a minute or two until wilted. Season and serve.

Chefs Note....
Edamame are delicious Asian soya beans.

Coconut Egg Curry

500 calories per serving

Ingredients

- 200g/7oz cauliflower florets
- 1 garlic clove, crushed
- 1 onion, chopped
- 75g/3oz green beans
- 2 tsp olive oil
- 1 tbsp tomato puree
- 200g/7oz tinned chopped tomatoes
- ½ tsp each turmeric, garam masala & ground coriander/cilantro
- 250ml/1 cup tinned coconut milk
- 3 large free-range hard-boiled eggs
- 1 tbsp freshly chopped coriander/cilantro
- Salt & pepper to taste

Method

1 First hard boil your eggs, peel and put to one side.

2 Gently sauté the garlic, onions & green beans in the olive oil for a few minutes until softened.

3 Stir through the tomato puree, tinned chopped tomatoes, dried spices & coconut milk until combined. Cut the eggs in half and place yolk side up, in the coconut milk. Gently cook until warmed through.

4 Meanwhile place the cauliflower florets in a food processor and pulse a few times until the cauliflower is the size of rice grains.

5 Place the 'rice' in a microwavable dish, cover and cook on full power for about 90 seconds or until it's piping hot.

6 Tip the 'rice' into a shallow bowl add the egg curry and serve with chopped coriander over the top.

Chefs Note....

Egg curry is very popular in Southern India where eggs are often a primary source of protein.

Fiery Pork & Brown Rice

515 calories per serving

Ingredients

- 50g/2oz brown rice
- 1 tbsp extra virgin olive oil
- 50g/2oz red onion
- 50g/2oz green beans, chopped
- 2 garlic cloves, crushed
- 1 red chilli, sliced
- 2 tbsp lime juice
- 2 tbsp fish sauce
- ½ tsp brown sugar
- 150g/5oz pork tenderloin, cubed
- 1 tbsp chopped corinader
- 50g/2oz spinach
- Salt & pepper to taste

Method

1 Cook the rice in salted boiling water until tender and drain.

2 Meanwhile heat up a frying pan with the olive oil and start sautéing the onions for a few minutes until softened.

3 Add the pork and while it's cooking combine the garlic cloves, chilli, lime juice, fish sauce and brown sugar to make a spicy, sweet & sour dressing.

4 When the pork is cooked, tip the drained rice into the pan and warm for a few minutes until everything is piping hot.

5 Add the spinach and stir for a few moments until it is gently wilted.

6 Tip the pork and rice into a shallow bowl, drizzle the dressing over the top and sprinkle with coriander.

Chefs Note....
Balance the chilli, lime and sugar to suit your own taste in the fiery Vietnamese dressing.

Fruity Giant Couscous

475 calories per serving

Ingredients

- 75g/3oz wholemeal couscous
- 500ml/2 cups vegetable stock
- 3 tbsp pomegranate seeds
- 2 tsp lemon juice
- 1 tbsp extra virgin olive oil
- 1 tbsp fresh mint, chopped
- 2 tbsp flat leaf parsley, chopped
- 50g/2oz carrot, grated
- 50g/2oz celery, sliced
- 50g/2oz feta cheese, crumbled
- 1 tbsp balsamic vinegar
- Salt & pepper to taste

Method

1 Put the couscous in a saucepan, cover and cook in boiling vegetable stock for about 6-8 minutes or until it's tender. (Add more vegetable stock if needed).

2 Once the couscous is ready, drain it and fluff with a fork. Combine with the pomegranate seeds, lemon juice, olive oil, mint and parsley.

3 Pile the grated carrot and sliced celery on top. Add the crumbled feta cheese and drizzle the balsamic vinegar over the cheese.

4 Season and serve.

Chefs Note....
Add as much balsamic vinegar as you like to this crunchy salad.

Cauliflower Rice & Pork

550 calories per serving

Ingredients

- ½ red onion, chopped
- 75g/3oz spinach
- 1 garlic clove, crushed
- 1 tbsp extra virgin olive oil
- 125g/4oz cherry tomatoes, chopped
- 1 tbsp sultanas
- 150g/5oz port tenderloin, cubed

- 2 tsp medium curry powder
- 2 tbsp coconut cream
- 2 tbsp flat leaf parsley, chopped
- 200g/7oz cauliflower florets
- 1 tbsp chopped coriander/cilantro
- Salt & pepper to taste

Method

1 Gently cook the onions, garlic, cherry tomatoes & sultanas in a frying pan with the olive oil. Sauté for a few minutes and then add the pork & curry powder (add a little more olive oil if needed).

2 Cook for a few minutes until the pork is cooked through then stir through the coconut cream, spinach and parsley to warm and wilt.

3 Meanwhile place the cauliflower florets in a food processor and pulse a few times until the cauliflower is the size of rice grains.

4 Place the 'rice' in a microwavable dish, cover and cook on full power for about 90 seconds minutes or until it's piping hot.

5 Tip the 'rice' into a shallow bowl. Serve the pork and vegetables over the top sprinkled with chopped coriander.

Chefs Note....
Prawns are also good in this simple spiced dish.

5

Super Simple

DESSERTS

Peanut Butter Pancakes

300 calories per serving

Ingredients

- 2 eggs
- 2 tbsp coconut milk
- 1 tbsp sugar free peanut butter
- 1 tbsp coconut flour
- 2 tsp coconut oil
- ½ tsp vanilla extract

Method

1 Place all the ingredients, except the coconut oil, in a blender and whizz until smooth.

2 Heat a little coconut oil in a small frying pan on a high heat. Pour in half the batter and fry until golden underneath (about 1 min if the pan is hot enough).

3 Flip and fry for a minute longer.

Chefs Note....
Greek yoghurt and berries makes a great addition to this super dessert.

Beetroot Brownie Bites

130 calories per serving

Ingredients

- 125g/4oz coconut flour
- 100g/3½oz cocoa nibs
- Pinch sea salt
- 1 tsp baking powder
- 1 tsp vanilla extract

- 2 tbsp coconut oil
- 1 tbsp water
- 1 tbsp honey
- 1 tbsp grated beetroot
- 2 tbsp almond butter, melted

Method

1 Preheat the oven to 180C/350F/Gas Mark 4.

2 Combine all the ingredients into a dough and form into 8-10 balls with your hands.

3 Lay out on a piece of baking parchment on a baking tray and cook for 20-25 minutes or until cooked through.

Chefs Note....

Use extra flour or water/oil as needed if you find the dough is too wet or dry during preparation.

Mini Mint Meringues

65 calories per serving

Ingredients

- 5 large egg whites
- 1 tsp stevia
- ¼ tsp sea salt
- 125g/4oz unsweetened coconut flakes
- 1 tsp finely chopped mint

Method

1 Use a mixer to whisk together the egg whites and stevia to form stiff peaks. Gently 'fold' in the salt, coconut flakes and finely chopped mint, using the minimum amount of folding to keep all the air in the egg white mixture. Cover and place in the refrigerator to chill for 30-40 minutes.

2 Preheat the oven to 180C/350F/Gas Mark 5.

3 Lay out a piece of baking parchment on an oven tray. Use a small ice cream scoop to make meringue mounds which you turn out onto the baking parchment. (Make sure each scoop is packed tight by pressing down with the palm of your hand on the filling when it is in the scoop).

4 Bake in a preheated oven for 9-12 minutes or until the meringues gently begin to brown.

Chefs Note....
The mint adds a little twist to this simple dessert but feel free to leave out. Delicious served with fresh berries.

Cocoa Cinnamon Cookies

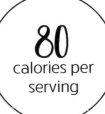

80 calories per serving

Ingredients

- 375g/13oz almond flour
- ½ tsp sea salt
- ¼ tsp baking soda
- 2 tsp ground cinnamon

- 100g/3½oz cocoa nibs
- 2 tsp vanilla extract
- 60ml/¼ cup coconut oil

Method

1 Mix together the flour, salt, baking powder, cinnamon and cocoa nibs.

2 In a separate bowl mix together the oil & vanilla and, when combined, mix the contents of each bowl together to make a ball of dough. Cover and leave to chill for about an hour.

3 Preheat the oven to 180C/350F/Gas Mark 4.

4 Roll out the dough onto a floured surface (use a little almond flour) until the dough is about 1cm/¼ inch thick. Use a small cookie cutter to make approx. 30 cookies (depending on the size of your cutter).

5 Place the cut cookies on baking parchment on a baking tray and cook in the preheated oven for 5-7 minutes or until they begin to gently brown. Take out of the oven and leave to cool on a rack.

Chefs Note....

Three cookies are appropriate for a dessert serving.

Blueberry Mousse

275 calories per serving

Ingredients

- 225g/8oz blueberries
- 1 tsp stevia
- ½ tsp vanilla extract
- 2 tbsp coconut oil

- 2 tbsp coconut butter
- 1 tbsp lemon juice
- 1 tsp grated coconut

Method

1 Rinse the blueberries and pat dry.

2 Very gently warm the coconut oil and butter together until combined.

3 Place all the ingredients, except the grated coconut, in a blender and whizz until smooth.

4 Pour into a small bowl and chill for a couple of hours until firm.

5 Sprinkle the grated coconut over the top to serve

Chefs Note....
A little chopped mint also makes a nice addition.

10
Low Cal
SMOOTHIES

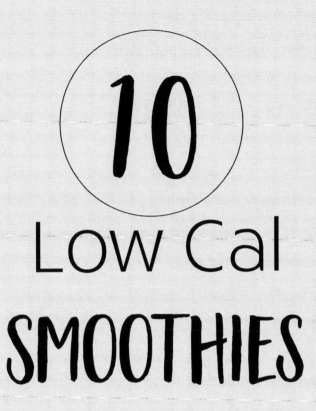

Time to try....
the
BLOOD SUGER
DIET

Double Berry Blast

95 calories per serving

Ingredients

- 40g/1½oz spinach
- 75g/3oz blueberries
- 75g/3oz blackberries
- Water

Method

1 Rinse the ingredients well.

2 Cut any thick green stalks off the spinach.

3 Add the fruit & vegetables to your blender. Make sure the ingredients do not go past the MAX line on your machine.

4 Add water, again being careful not to exceed the MAX line.

5 Blend until smooth.

Chefs Note....
Any mix of soft berries will work for this simple smoothie. If it's a little sharp add 1 tsp honey (21 calories).

Pear Pepper Juice

Ingredients

- 75g/3oz spinach
- 1 medium yellow pepper
- 75g/3oz ripe pear
- Water

Method

1 Rinse the ingredients well.

2 Remove any thick stalks from the spinach.

3 De-seed and core the yellow pepper & pear.

4 Add the fruit & spinach to your blender. Make sure the ingredients do not go past the MAX line on your machine.

5 Add water, again being careful not to exceed the MAX line.

6 Blend until smooth.

Chefs Note....
Any coloured sweet pepper will work for this juice (not green though as it has a bitter taste).

Blueberry Broccolini

99 calories per serving

Ingredients

- 75g/3oz tenderstem broccoli/broccolini
- 75g/3oz blueberries
- 1 tsp honey
- Water

Method

1 Rinse the ingredients well.

2 Cut any thick woody ends off the broccoli.

3 Add the fruit, vegetables and honey to your blender. Make sure the ingredients do not go past the MAX line on your machine.

4 Add water, again being careful not to exceed the MAX line.

5 Blend until smooth.

Chefs Note....
Purple sprouting broccoli is a lovely tenderstem broccoli to use when it's in season.

Cranberry & Broccoli Mint Juice

132 calories per serving

Ingredients

- 125g/4oz cranberries
- 75g/3oz broccoli florets
- 1 tbsp chopped mint
- 1 tbsp pumpkin seeds
- Water

Method

1 Rinse the ingredients well.

2 Add the fruit, vegetables, mint & pumpkin seeds to your blender. Make sure the ingredients do not go past the MAX line on your machine.

3 Add water, again being careful not to exceed the MAX line.

4 Blend until smooth.

Chefs Note....
Cranberries are thought to have a positive effect on the immune system.

Berry Almond Milk Smoothie

98 calories per serving

Ingredients

- 40g/1½oz blackberries
- 40g/1½oz raspberries
- 100ml/3½floz unsweetened almond milk
- Water

Method

1 Rinse the ingredients well.

2 Add the fruit & almond milk to your blender. Make sure the ingredients do not go past the MAX line on your machine.

3 Add water, again being careful not to exceed the MAX line.

4 Blend until smooth.

Chefs Note....
Adjust the quantity of water to get the consistency you prefer.

Coconut Green Smoothie

115 calories per serving

Ingredients

- 75g/3oz spinach
- 400ml/14floz coconut water
- 1 tsp honey
- Handful of ice cubes (optional)

Method

1 Rinse the spinach well and cut off any thick stalks.

2 Add the spinach, honey & coconut water to your blender. Make sure the ingredients do not go past the MAX line on your machine. (If you are adding ice cubes you may need to use a little less coconut water).

3 Blend until smooth.

Chefs Note....
It's best to use unsweetened 100% coconut water.

Green Cauliflower Smoothie

97 calories per serving

Ingredients

- 75g/3oz cauliflower florets
- 75g/3oz watercress
- 100ml/3½floz unsweetened almond milk
- 1 tsp honey
- Water

Method

1 Rinse the ingredients well.

2 Add the cauliflower, watercress, honey & almond milk to your blender. Make sure the ingredients do not go past the MAX line on your machine.

3 Add water, again being careful not to exceed the MAX line.

4 Blend until smooth.

Chefs Note....
Cauliflower is a surprisingly good source of Vitamin C.

Almond Carrot Smoothie

195
calories per serving

Ingredients

- 50g/2oz spinach
- 125g/4oz carrots
- 200ml/7floz unsweetened almond milk
- 1 tbsp ground almonds
- Water

Method

1 Rinse the ingredients well.

2 Cut any thick green stalks off the spinach.

3 Top & tail the carrots, no need to peel.

4 Add the vegetables, almond milk & ground almonds to your blender. Make sure the ingredients do not go past the MAX line on your machine.

5 Add a little water if needed to take it up to the MAX line.

6 Blend until smooth.

Chefs Note....
The ground almonds help create a thick base for this double nut smoothie.

Sunshine Radish Smoothie

189 calories per serving

Ingredients

- 50g/2oz spinach
- 200g/7oz pink grapefruit
- 125g/4oz radishes
- 200ml/7floz unsweetened almond milk
- Water

Method

1 Rinse the ingredients well.

2 Cut any thick green stalks off the spinach.

3 Peel and de-seed the grapefruit

4 Nip the tops of the radishes.

5 Add the fruit, vegetables & almond milk to your blender. Make sure the ingredients do not go past the MAX line on your machine.

6 Add a little water if needed to take it up to the MAX line.

7 Blend until smooth.

Chefs Note....
Any type of grapefruit is fine to use but pink will give you the best result.

Super Green Cucumber Juice

110 calories per serving

Ingredients

- 50g/2oz spinach
- ½ cucumber
- 2 tbsp lemon juice
- 1 tbsp flax seed
- Water

Method

1 Rinse the ingredients well.

2 Cut any thick green stalks off the spinach.

3 Nip the end of the cucumber but don't bother peeling it.

4 Add the spinach, cucumber, lemon juice & flax seed to your blender. Make sure the ingredients do not go past the MAX line on your machine.

5 Add water, again being careful not to exceed the MAX line.

6 Blend until smooth.

Chefs Note....
Cucumbers contain vitamin K, B vitamins, copper, potassium, vitamin C, and manganese.

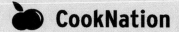 **CookNation**

Other
CookNation
titles

If you enjoyed *'Time to try... the BLOOD SUGAR DIET'* you may also enjoy other books from CookNation including:

'Time to try... the FAST DIET'

'Time to try...VEGAN'

and the extensive calorie counted *'Skinny'* range of books.

To browse the full catalogue visit
www.bellmackenzie.com

Printed in Great Britain
by Amazon